Dr Clara J. Combest

"Berberine Breakthrough

Unlocking the Power of Herbal Medicine for Metabolic Health and Beyond."

Disclaimer

Contents

Berberine Breakthrough

Overview of berberine

A naturally occurring substance called berberine is obtained from a variety of plants, mainly those in the genus Berberis. It is a yellow alkaloid that has been utilized for many years in Ayurvedic and traditional Chinese medicine. Berberine has a broad variety of medicinal benefits, including actions that are antibacterial, anti-inflammatory, antioxidant, and anti-diabetic. Due to its possible health advantages and capacity to modify a number of biochemical processes in the human body, it has received a great deal of interest lately.

Several plant species, including Chinese goldthread (Coptis chinensis), barberry (Berberis vulgaris), Oregon grape (Berberis aquifolium), and goldenseal (Hydrastis canadensis), contain berberine. These plants' rhizomes, bark, stalks, roots, and stems are used to extract the chemical. Traditional medicine has traditionally used berberine to treat a variety of ailments, including infections, diabetes, cardiovascular disease, and gastrointestinal problems.

Berberine has a bicyclic structure made up of isoquinoline rings in its chemical makeup. It is well recognized for its capacity to engage with a variety of bodily targets, such as enzymes, receptors, and signaling cascades. Berberine exerts its therapeutic effects and adds to its wide variety of health advantages via these interactions.

Berberine has been the subject of promising research in a number of fields, including the control of blood sugar levels, enhancement of lipid profiles, reduction of inflammation, improvement of gastrointestinal health, and support of cardiovascular health. Berberine is a possible contender for treating infections since it has also shown antibacterial capabilities against bacteria, fungi, and viruses.

It is crucial to think about the safety and possible adverse effects of berberine, as with any chemical. Although typically well-tolerated, berberine may have certain negative effects and interact with a few drugs when used in large dosages or for an extended period of time. Before utilizing berberine as a dietary supplement or for therapeutic effects, it is essential to speak with a healthcare provider.

Berberine has a long history, especially in the conventional medicinal procedures of ancient societies. Various civilizations have known and used the therapeutic benefits of berberine-rich plants for ages, including those in China and India.

Herbs containing berberine, such as Rhizoma coptidis (goldenthread) and Coptis chinensis (Chinese goldthread), have been widely utilized in traditional Chinese medicine. The "Shennong Ben Cao Jing" (Divine Farmer's Materia Medica), which dates back to the Han era (206 BCE–220 CE), has descriptions of these plants. Herbs high in berberine have been used in traditional Chinese medicine to treat infections, inflammation, and digestive problems.

Berberine-containing plants like Berberis aristata (Indian barberry) and Berberis vulgaris (barberry) have been used for their medicinal properties in Ayurvedic medicine, the age-old Indian healing system. These plants are mentioned in Ayurvedic writings including the "Charaka Samhita" and the "Sushruta Samhita" for their use in treating urinary problems, skin conditions, and digestive problems.

The historical relevance of berberine extends beyond Eastern medicine. Native American tribes including the Cherokee, Iroquois, and Cheyenne were aware of the therapeutic benefits of herbs like Hydrastis canadensis (goldenseal) that contain berberine. These tribes used goldenseal for a variety of conditions, such as painful eyes, stomach problems, and wound healing.

Berberine's effectiveness as a medicine has been shown by its historical usage and acknowledgment. Ancient civilizations' collective wisdom and experience opened the path for contemporary science to investigate the pharmacological characteristics and possible health advantages of berberine.

To comprehend its methods of action and potential therapeutic uses, berberine is still a topic of intense scientific investigation today. The historical importance of berberine as a folk cure has influenced its appeal in modern herbal medicine and encouraged more research into its potential as a useful medicinal substance.

Obtaining Berberine

The main sources of berberine are the rhizomes, stems, roots, and bark of numerous plants. It is known that a number of plant species contain significant levels of berberine. The following are some typical berberine sources:

1. Chinese goldthread, Coptis chinensis

The herbaceous perennial plant Coptis chinensis, sometimes referred to as Chinese goldthread, is significant in traditional Chinese medicine. It is indigenous to East Asia, namely China. The vivid golden hue of its rhizomes, which resemble threads, is whence Chinese goldthread gets its name.

Since ancient times, traditional Chinese herbal treatments have utilized the Coptis chinensis rhizomes due to their valuable therapeutic qualities. They have a large quantity of berberine, which is what gives them many of its medicinal properties.

Coptis chinensis is referred to as Huang Lian in conventional Chinese medicine. Its traditional categorization based on its energy qualities places it in the "cold" category of herbs. Huang Lian has a bitter flavor and is known for its ability to remove heat and cleanse the body. It is said to have a cooling impact on the body, treating ailments brought on by overheating and inflammation.

Traditional treatments for Coptis chinensis have included gastrointestinal problems, infections, inflammation, and liver-related problems. Due to its medicinal properties, it is often used in herbal formulations or given as a standalone plant.

One of the plant's main bioactive ingredients, berberine, is thought to be present in Coptis chinensis. The potential health advantages of berberine, including its antibacterial, anti-inflammatory, and blood sugar-regulating capabilities, have been thoroughly explored. It has been shown to interact with a variety of molecular targets in the body, which helps explain the wide range of pharmacological effects it has.

Coptis chinensis has been used in cooking techniques in addition to its medical use. The rhizomes' bright yellow hue makes them sometimes used as a natural food color.

The plant Coptis chinensis is still valued in traditional Chinese medicine and is receiving more attention in contemporary scientific studies. Its reputation as a useful medicinal herb has been aided by research into its active ingredients, especially berberine.

2. Barberry, Berberis vulgaris

The shrub Berberis vulgaris, sometimes called barberry, is indigenous to Europe, Africa, and Asia. It is a member of the Berberidaceae family and has long been valued for its therapeutic benefits.

A notable feature of barberry is its spiky branches and bunches of vivid red berries. Berberine, one of the plant's most noteworthy components, is one of the many bioactive substances it contains.

Traditional medical practices, such as Ayurveda, Chinese medicine, and European herbal traditions, have long used Berberis vulgaris. Its berries, roots, and bark are used for their medicinal properties.

The herb Berberis vulgaris has been used to treat a range of medical illnesses, including issues with the liver, the digestive system, and the urinary system. It is renowned for its bitter flavor, which is said to stimulate the digestive system and enhance the functioning of the liver.

One of the primary therapeutic components of barberry is thought to be its berberine concentration. A naturally occurring alkaloid called berberine has a wide range of antimicrobial activities, including actions against viruses, fungi, and bacteria. The possibility of it preventing infections and boosting immune system function has been well-researched.

Barberry also has culinary purposes in addition to its medical ones. The berries of Berberis vulgaris are prized for their tart flavor and are sometimes used in jam, jelly, and herbal tea preparations.

Despite the fact that barberry has a long history of traditional usage, it should only be consumed or used as a supplement when under adequate medical supervision. Before utilizing barberry for therapeutic reasons, as with any other medicinal plant, a healthcare practitioner should be consulted.

The scientific study continues to be done on barberry (Berberis vulgaris), which is still known for its possible health advantages. In traditional and herbal medical systems, it is regarded as a beneficial plant because of its bioactive components, which include berberine.

3. Goldenseal, Hydrastis canadensis

The perennial plant Hydrastis canadensis, sometimes referred to as goldenseal, is indigenous to eastern North America. It has a long history of usage in both Western herbal medicine and Native American herbal medicine, giving it a reputation as a useful medicinal plant.

The roots and stems of goldenseal are brilliant yellow and have hairs on them. The therapeutic qualities of Hydrastis canadensis are mostly found in its roots and rhizomes.

Goldenseal has been used in traditional medicine for a variety of causes. It has been used as a digestive aid, enhancing appetite and promoting good digestion. It is well-recognized for its bitter taste. As a mouthwash for dental health, as a wash for eye irritations, and as a topical treatment for skin disorders, goldenseal has also been utilized.

Berberine is one of the prominent ingredients in goldenseal. The bioactive alkaloid berberine is what gives goldenseal its distinctively yellow hue. It is well recognized for its antibacterial qualities, which include action against certain parasites, fungi, and bacteria. Due to this, goldenseal is a well-liked remedy for infections, especially those that impact the digestive and respiratory systems.

Recent media emphasis on goldenseal has raised questions about its sustainability and protection. Wild goldenseal populations have decreased as a result of overharvesting and habitat destruction. The plant is now categorized as a threatened species in certain areas as a consequence. It's crucial to get goldenseal items from reliable vendors that use sustainable harvesting techniques or take into account herbs with comparable qualities.

Although goldenseal is still prized in herbal therapy, it is crucial to speak with a doctor before taking goldenseal supplements or products, particularly at large dosages or for a long time. Goldenseal may interact with certain drugs, therefore it's crucial to address any possible interactions with a healthcare professional.

Hydrostis canadensis, sometimes known as goldenseal, is still a crucial plant in conventional and herbal therapy. The plant is now recognized as a medicinal herb with possible health advantages as a result of historical usage and continuing scientific investigation.

4. Oregon grapes, Mahonia aquifolium

The evergreen shrub Mahonia aquifolium, sometimes known as the Oregon grape, is a native of western North America. It bears characteristics with other Berberis species like barberry and is a member of the Berberidaceae family. The Oregon grape has a long history of usage in both Native American and Western herbal medicine and is highly prized for its therapeutic qualities.

The holly-like leaves and clusters of tiny yellow blossoms eventually turn into dark blue berries that distinguish the Oregon grape. Mahonia aquifolium's rhizomes, bark, and roots are used for their medicinal properties.

The Oregon grape has been used for a number of health issues in conventional Native American medicine. As a digestive tonic, it has been used to improve normal digestion and increase appetite. The plant has historically been used to treat infections, skin conditions, and urinary tract problems. It is also recognized for its antibacterial capabilities.

Berberine, a significant bioactive component of Oregon grape, is what gives it many of its medicinal properties. An alkaloid with antibacterial, anti-inflammatory, and antioxidant effects is berberine. It supports the Oregon grape's standing as an important therapeutic plant.

Due to their comparable berberine content and therapeutic benefits, Oregon grape and goldenseal (Hydrastis canadensis) are often substituted in Western herbal medicine. It is regarded as a bitter herb and is used to enhance liver health, stimulate digestive processes, and encourage good skin.

There are many ways to consume Oregon grapes, including extracts, tinctures, and topical solutions. The Oregon grape should only be taken under the supervision of a healthcare provider since, like other berberine-rich plants, it may interfere with certain medicines.

Sustainable harvesting methods and cultivation efforts are urged to protect the preservation of the Oregon grape and its natural habitats due to its popularity and rising demand.

Mahonia aquifolium, sometimes known as the Oregon grape, is still being studied by scientists because of its possible health advantages. Its reputation as a potent herbal cure is influenced by both its historical usage in traditional medicine and continuing research.

5. Heart-leaved moonseed, Tinospora cordifolia

The climbing shrub Tinospora cordifolia, sometimes called heart-leaved moonseed or Giloy, is indigenous to Southeast Asia and India. In Ayurvedic medicine, India's ancient medical system, it is of utmost importance.

The heart-shaped leaves that decorate the vines of heart-leaved moonseed give it its name. The plant has long been revered in Ayurveda for its wide variety of health advantages and for its medicinal capabilities.

Tinospora cordifolia is referred to as Giloy or Guduchi in Ayurvedic medicine. It is a rasayana, a kind of plant said to support general health and long life and is regarded as a multipurpose herb.

Historically, giloy has been used to treat a number of medical issues. It is often used as an immunomodulator, boosting the body's defense mechanisms and fostering infection resistance. Additionally, it is renowned for its adaptogenic qualities, which aid the body in adjusting to both physical and mental stress.

Tinospora cordifolia stems, leaves, and roots are used for their therapeutic qualities. Typically, they are transformed into powders, decoctions, and herbal formulations, among other forms.

Heart-leaved moonseed contains a number of important bioactive substances, including a class of chemicals known as bitter principles. Alkaloids and diterpenoids are two bitter compounds that support the herb's medicinal properties.

For its possible health advantages, Tinospora cordifolia has been the subject of substantial research. Antioxidant, anti-inflammatory, and antibacterial properties are thought to exist in it. Additionally, it has hepatoprotective qualities that promote liver health and facilitates the detoxification process.

To increase the effectiveness of other herbs and encourage their absorption and assimilation in the body, giloy is often utilized in Ayurvedic formulations. It is regarded as a useful plant for boosting vigor and fostering general well-being.

Before taking Tinospora cordifolia or any other herbal supplement for therapeutic reasons, as with any herbal medicine, it is advised to speak with a licensed Ayurvedic practitioner or healthcare expert.

Tinospora cordifolia, often known as heart-leaved moonseed, is still held in high respect in Ayurvedic medicine for its possible health advantages. Its reputation as a useful medicinal herb is influenced by both its historical usage and current scientific studies.

Berberine's traditional uses

Different civilizations have traditionally used berberine, a bioactive substance found in several plants including Coptis chinensis (Chinese goldthread), Berberis vulgaris (barberry), and Berberis aristata (Indian barberry).

Here are a few of its customary applications:

1. Gastrointestinal Health: Berberine, a bioactive chemical present in a number of plants, has long been utilized to enhance gastrointestinal health. It is said to help regular bowel motions, improve healthy digestion, and reduce gastrointestinal pain. Its usage in conventional medical systems implies that it has the ability to treat digestive problems and preserve gastrointestinal health. The processes behind berberine's impact on digestive health are still being studied in depth.

2. Infections and Immune Support: Berberine, which is present in a number of plants, including Coptis chinensis, Berberis vulgaris, and Berberis aristata, has long been used to enhance the immune system and fight infections. It is effective in treating different illnesses because it has antibacterial characteristics that are effective against bacteria, fungi, and parasites. The immune system is thought to be strengthened by berberine, which also helps the body defend itself against viruses. Investigation into its potential for promoting immunological health and warding off infections is still ongoing.

3. Liver Health: Berberine has long been utilized to maintain the health of the liver. It is said to contain hepatoprotective qualities that support liver health and the body's detoxification processes. Current research indicates that berberine may have advantageous effects on lipid metabolism, oxidative stress, and liver enzymes, which add to its potential to improve liver health.

4. Blood Sugar control: Berberine's possible effects on blood sugar control have been researched. Berberine may maintain healthy blood sugar levels by enhancing insulin sensitivity and enhancing glucose metabolism, according to research. Additionally, it could prevent several liver enzymes from producing glucose. However, before using berberine or any other supplement for blood sugar control, particularly for those with pre-existing medical issues or those taking drugs that alter blood sugar levels, it is very important to speak with a health professionals.

5. Skin Disorders: Berberine, which is present in a number of plants including Coptis chinensis (Chinese goldthread), Berberis vulgaris (barberry), and Berberis aristata (Indian barberry), has long been used to treat a number of skin disorders. It has become a well-liked option for treating infections, rashes, and acne because of its possible antibacterial and anti-inflammatory effects. Berberine's historic usage in creating better skin may be aided by its ability to fight microbial overgrowth and reduce inflammation.

6. Respiratory health: Traditional uses for berberine, a bioactive chemical present in several plants, include supporting respiratory health. It is said to have qualities that might help ease the symptoms of coughs, sore throats, and respiratory infections. The potential advantages of berberine for respiratory health are still being investigated through ongoing studies.

7. Effects on Inflammation: Berberine, a bioactive chemical present in a variety of plants, has been identified for its ability to reduce inflammation. It has long been used to treat inflammatory diseases such as inflammatory bowel disease and arthritis. The ways in which berberine may control inflammatory responses in the body are now the subject of scientific investigation. It has the potential to be an effective natural medicine for enhancing general health and well-being due to its anti-inflammatory characteristics.

Berberine Breakthrough

It's important to remember that traditional berberine applications differ between cultures and across particular plant sources. Traditional knowledge of berberine has helped it gain recognition as a beneficial therapeutic substance, and continuing scientific study is still looking into its possible health advantages.

Berberine's chemical makeup and properties

Alkaloids are a class of bioactive compounds that includes berberine. Coptis chinensis (Chinese goldthread), Berberis vulgaris (barberry), Berberis aristata (Indian barberry), and other plants all contain it. The following are some significant characteristics of its chemical makeup:

1. The molecular makeup of berberine

The intricate arrangement of atoms that make up the molecular structure of berberine gives it its distinct chemical makeup. As an isoquinoline alkaloid, which is a sort of naturally occurring substance present in many plant species, berberine is categorized.

Berberine is made up of the atoms carbon (C), hydrogen (H), nitrogen (N), and oxygen (O) at the molecular level. Its molecular structure is $C_{20}H_{18}NO_4^+$.

The isoquinoline bicyclic ring system makes up the primary structure of berberine. It has two fused rings: a benzene ring, which is bigger, and a pyridine ring, which is smaller. The primary scaffold of the molecule is the isoquinoline core.

The isoquinoline core is surrounded by a number of side chains and functional groups. Methoxy groups ($-OCH_3$) and hydroxyl groups ($-OH$) at certain locations within the structure are examples of these.

Additionally, berberine may be found in its salt form, berberine chloride or berberine sulfate, in which the ion chloride or sulfate is joined to the molecule of berberine. The stability and solubility of berberine in diverse applications are aided by these salt forms.

The biological actions and pharmacological effects of berberine are significantly influenced by its distinctive molecular structure. It enables berberine to interact with certain molecular targets in the body, affecting different physiological processes and displaying a variety of possible health advantages.

Studying berberine's features, modes of action, and possible uses in science and medicine requires an understanding of the compound's molecular structure.

2. Berberine's Physicochemical Characteristics

The natural substance berberine has unique physicochemical features that contribute to its medical and pharmacological qualities. The following are some of the berberine's prominent physicochemical characteristics:

Berberine is a chemical compound with the molecular formula $C_{20}H_{18}NO_4^+$. The configuration and sorts of atoms found in a single molecule of berberine are represented by this formula.

Molecular Weight: Berberine has a molecular weight of around 336.37 g/mol. The atomic weights of every atom in the molecule are added together to compute it.

Berberine is very weakly soluble in water. In organic solvents like ethanol and methanol, it dissolves more easily. Temperature, pH, and the presence of other chemicals may all have an impact on how soluble berberine is.

Melting Point: Berberine is said to have a melting point between 145 and 148 degrees Celsius. The temperature at which a material transitions from a solid to a liquid state is known as the melting point.

Berberine often takes the form of a brilliant yellow, orange-yellow, or yellow crystalline powder. Its hue, which is a result of its chemical composition, makes it useful as a natural dye.

pH Sensitivity: Berberine's properties are pH-dependent. In alkaline circumstances, it is less soluble and more soluble in acidic settings. The solubility and stability of berberine may be impacted by the pH of a solution.

Stability: Berberine is unstable in the presence of heat, light, and oxidizing agents. Under these circumstances, it may degrade, which would reduce its efficacy and shorten its shelf life. The stability of goods containing berberine must be maintained by proper formulation and storage methods.

These physicochemical characteristics of berberine affect its solubility, bioavailability, formulation, and stability. For creating suitable dosage forms, enhancing delivery methods, and assuring the quality and efficiency of berberine-based products in pharmaceutical and therapeutic applications, it is crucial to comprehend these features.

3. Pharmacokinetics effects of berberine

The study of how a material, such as a medicine or a molecule, is absorbed, distributed, metabolized, and removed by the body is known as pharmacokinetics. In order to determine a substance's efficacy, dose, and possible interactions with other medications or chemicals, it is essential to understand its pharmacokinetics.

The pharmacokinetics of the bioactive substance berberine, which is present in a number of plants, including Coptis chinensis (Chinese goldthread), Berberis vulgaris (barberry), and Berberis aristata (Indian barberry), may be summed up as follows:

Absorption: Berberine is normally used orally, and because of its weak solubility and low bioavailability, its absorption from the gastrointestinal system may be restricted. Its absorption may be influenced by factors including food consumption and the presence of other drugs. It has been investigated how to improve berberine absorption by co-administering it with substances like piperine.

Distribution: The liver, kidneys, intestines, skin, and other tissues and organs are thought to be among the places where berberine is abundantly distributed. It may partially pass the blood-brain barrier.

Metabolism: Berberine is extensively metabolized in the liver, mainly in phase I metabolism, which is regulated by cytochrome P450 enzymes. Dihydroberberine and berberrubine are two of berberine's main metabolites. Compared to the original molecule, these metabolites may have distinct pharmacological actions.

Elimination: Berberine and its metabolites are mostly eliminated via the biliary system, with a little amount ending up in the urine. Berberine has a variable elimination half-life and may be reabsorbed from the intestines after being discharged into bile. It may also be prone to enterohepatic circulation.

It is important to remember that a number of variables, including the dose form, individual differences in metabolism, and possible medication interactions, might affect the pharmacokinetics of berberine. Furthermore, berberine's pharmacokinetics may vary depending on the precise plant source and formulation employed.

To improve berberine administration and expand its therapeutic potential, research on its pharmacokinetics is continuing. It is essential to know how berberine is absorbed, transported, metabolized, and removed in order to choose the right dose regimen, maximize its positive benefits, and reduce any hazards.

4. Pharmaceutical effects of berberine

Berberine, a naturally occurring chemical present in many plants, has a variety of pharmacodynamic characteristics, which pertain to its interactions with biological targets and the effects on the body that arise. The following are some significant facets of berberine's pharmacodynamics:

Molecular Targets: The body's enzymes, receptors, and signaling pathways are only a few of the many molecules that berberine interacts with. AMP-activated protein kinase (AMPK), protein kinase B (Akt), nuclear factor kappa B (NF-B), and numerous metabolic enzymes involved in glucose and lipid metabolism are a few of the significant targets.

Glucose Regulation: Berberine has been shown to have considerable impacts on the metabolism of glucose. It may increase insulin sensitivity, boost cellular absorption of glucose, reduce hepatic glucose synthesis, and modify a number of signaling pathways involved in glucose management. These activities support its potential advantages in controlling blood sugar levels.

Lipid Metabolism: Berberine may have an effect on lipid metabolism by lowering the production of cholesterol and triglycerides, preventing the absorption of dietary fats, and encouraging the liver's breakdown of lipids. Its potential utility in treating lipid problems and promoting cardiovascular health may be influenced by these actions.

Anti-inflammatory Activity: Berberine inhibits pro-inflammatory cytokines and enzymes that are involved in the inflammatory response, exhibiting anti-inflammatory characteristics. A crucial regulator of inflammation, NF-B, can be modulated with the aid of this. The potential advantages of berberine in illnesses linked to chronic inflammation may be influenced by this anti-inflammatory impact.

Antimicrobial Effects: Broad-spectrum antimicrobial effects of berberine include action against bacteria, fungi, parasites, and viruses. It may harm microbial DNA replication, impede microbial enzymes, and damage microbial cell membranes. Berberine is a useful natural antibiotic due to its antibacterial characteristics.

Antioxidant Activity: Berberine's antioxidant benefits are shown through scavenging free radicals and lowering oxidative stress. It may boost endogenous antioxidant enzyme activity and reduce the production of reactive oxygen species. Its potential advantages in preventing cellular damage and promoting general health may be attributed to its antioxidant action.

Effects on Cancer: Laboratory tests have shown that berberine may be able to prevent the development and division of cancer cells. It has the ability to stop the cell cycle, encourage apoptosis (planned cell death), and prevent angiogenesis (the growth of new blood vessels). Although further study is required, these findings point to a possible role for berberine in the treatment and prevention of cancer.

The pharmacodynamics of berberine might change based on the precise dose, formulation, and individual characteristics, it is crucial to note. Furthermore, research is currently being done to determine the specific mechanisms of action for these effects. Before utilizing berberine or products containing berberine for certain health issues, it is recommended that you speak with a healthcare provider.

Benefits of Berberine for Health

The natural substance berberine has attracted a lot of interest recently because of its conceivable health advantages. Several plants, including barberry, goldenseal, Chinese goldthread, and Oregon grape, contain this bioactive alkaloid. Traditional medical practices like Ayurveda and traditional Chinese medicine have long used berberine. In this article, we shall examine Berberine's documented health advantages.

Blood sugar control

The capacity of berberine to control blood sugar is one of its most well-known advantages. Berberine has been shown in several trials to increase glucose metabolism, decrease fasting blood sugar levels, and improve insulin sensitivity. It causes the AMP-activated protein kinase (AMPK) enzyme to become active, aiding in the regulation of cellular energy balance. Berberine increases glucose absorption and utilization in cells by activating AMPK, enhancing insulin sensitivity, and lowering blood sugar levels as a result.

Weight Control

Additionally, berberine has shown promise in assisting with weight control. It may help with weight loss, body mass index (BMI), and waist circumference reduction. This is accomplished through berberine's regulation of metabolism, enhancement of fat oxidation, and inhibition of fat cell development. Berberine has also been shown to lessen hunger and food intake, which may help with weight reduction attempts.

Heart and Vascular Health

There are several advantages of berberine for cardiovascular health. It has been shown to raise HDL cholesterol (the "good" cholesterol) while decreasing total cholesterol, LDL cholesterol (the "bad" cholesterol), and triglyceride levels. This is accomplished through berberine's inhibition of PCSK9, an enzyme involved in the control of cholesterol. Berberine may help lessen the risk of heart disease and enhance general cardiovascular health by lowering cholesterol levels and lipid profiles.

Properties that Reduce Inflammation

Numerous diseases, such as cancer, diabetes, and cardiovascular disease, are linked to chronic inflammation. Berberine has been shown to have anti-inflammatory activities and to prevent the synthesis of inflammatory enzymes and cytokines. Berberine may help prevent or treat chronic inflammatory illnesses by lowering inflammation.

Bowel Health

The health of the gut has been proven to benefit from berberine. Encouraging the development of helpful bacteria and restraining the growth of harmful bacteria, may modify the gut microbiota. In order to keep the gut lining in good condition and stop toxins from entering the circulation, berberine is also helpful. Berberine enhances immunological and digestive health by encouraging a balanced gut microbiota and gut barrier function.

Biological Activity

Broad-spectrum antibacterial action is shown by berberine against a variety of pathogens, including bacteria, viruses, fungi, and parasites. It can stop microorganisms including Helicobacter pylori, Escherichia coli, and Staphylococcus aureus from multiplying and growing. In addition, berberine has antiviral properties against viruses including HIV, hepatitis B, and influenza. Its antifungal qualities work against Candida species, whereas Giardia lamblia and other protozoa have been shown to be resistant to its antiparasitic actions. Because of its antibacterial properties, berberine is an effective natural antibiotic.

hepatic health

Berberine maintains liver health and protects against liver damage since it contains hepatoprotective qualities. It has been shown to lessen the buildup of liver fat, promote liver function, and strengthen the body's natural antioxidant defenses. Berberine produces these results by raising AMPK, lowering oxidative stress, and controlling hepatic lipid metabolism. Berberine is advantageous for those with non-alcoholic fatty liver disease (NAFLD) and other liver diseases because of its liver-protective qualities.

Effects on Neuroprotection

Recent studies indicate that berberine may have neuroprotective properties and may be advantageous for brain health. It has been discovered to guard against neurodegenerative disorders including Alzheimer's and Parkinson's and can pass the blood-brain barrier. In the brain, berberine has anti-oxidant, anti-inflammatory, and anti-apoptotic (anti-cell death) characteristics that support its neuroprotective benefits.

Potential to combat cancer

Berberine has the potential as a natural cancer therapy and preventative agent. According to studies, berberine may stop the development and division of a variety of cancer cells, including those that are found in the liver, breast, colon, lung, and prostate. Berberine inhibits angiogenesis (the creation of new blood vessels that enable tumor growth), induces cell cycle arrest, and promotes apoptosis in order to exercise its anti-cancer actions.

Mindfulness and Mood
The effects of berberine on mood disorders and mental health have been researched. Berberine may have antidepressant and anxiolytic (anti-anxiety) properties, according to preliminary research. It is thought to have an impact on neurotransmitters that are important for controlling mood and emotions, such as serotonin and dopamine. To completely comprehend the effect of berberine on mental health, further study is required.

As a natural substance, berberine has a variety of possible health advantages. It is a versatile and useful natural remedy because of its capacity to control blood sugar, assist with weight management, improve cardiovascular health, reduce inflammation, promote gut health, display antimicrobial properties, protect the liver, show neuroprotective effects, possibly inhibit cancer growth, and have an impact on mental health. It is crucial to remember that more study is still required to completely comprehend its mechanisms of action, define the ideal dose, and assess its long-term safety. Before beginning berberine supplementation, like with any other supplement or natural treatment, it is advised to speak with a healthcare provider, particularly if you have any underlying medical concerns or are taking other drugs.

Systems of action

The exact methods by which a chemical causes its effects on the body are referred to as its mechanisms of action. Tinospora cordifolia, commonly known as heart-leaved moonseed or giloy, has a wide variety of health advantages, which have been the subject of numerous explanations. In order to shed light on the underlying mechanisms that contribute to Tinospora cordifolia's medicinal properties, this article will examine some of its main methods of action.

1. Pathways for Cellular Signaling

Because of its many medicinal benefits, berberine, a naturally occurring chemical present in many plants, particularly Berberis species, has drawn a lot of interest. Through the modification of cellular signaling pathways, berberine is able to have an impact on the body in a number of ways. These pathways have a significant impact on both general health and disease states by controlling a number of cellular activities. Here, we'll look at a few of the important cellular signaling pathways that berberine targets.

AMP-activated protein kinase (AMPK) pathway: The AMP-activated protein kinase (AMPK) pathway is a key player in controlling how cells use their energy. It has been shown that berberine activates AMPK, increasing glucose absorption, enhancing fatty acid oxidation, and enhancing mitochondrial activity. The promotion of energy balance is advantageous in situations including obesity, type 2 diabetes, and metabolic syndrome because of berberine's activation of the AMPK pathway.

Insulin signaling pathway: Berberine has been demonstrated to enhance insulin sensitivity and glucose homeostasis through the insulin signaling system. By boosting insulin receptor phosphorylation and subsequent signaling cascades, it stimulates the insulin signaling system. This results in greater absorption of glucose enhanced glycemic management, and decreased insulin resistance. In the setting of insulin resistance and type 2 diabetes, berberine's modulation of the insulin signaling pathway is especially pertinent.

Nuclear factor kappa B (NF-κB) pathway: The nuclear factor kappa B (NF-B) pathway is a transcription factor that controls immunological and inflammatory responses. It has been shown that berberine inhibits NF-B activation, which results in less pro-inflammatory cytokine production and the regulation of inflammatory pathways. In diseases like inflammatory bowel disease and rheumatoid arthritis, which are characterized by persistent inflammation, berberine's anti-inflammatory action is important.

Mitogen-activated protein kinase (MAPK) pathways: MAPK pathways are essential for cell division, proliferation, and death. The extracellular signal-regulated kinase (ERK), c-Jun N-terminal kinase (JNK), and p38 MAPK pathways are only a few of the MAPK pathways that berberine may influence. Berberine may affect cell proliferation, death, and inflammatory reactions by controlling MAPK signaling.

Wnt/-catenin pathway: The Wnt/-catenin pathway plays a role in biological functions such as tissue regeneration, cell proliferation, and development. The Wnt/-catenin pathway has been demonstrated to be inhibited by berberine, which may have effects on how cell division and proliferation are managed. The Wnt/-catenin pathway is modulated by berberine, which may be important in diseases like cancer where aberrant Wnt signaling is seen.

Akt/mTOR pathway: The Akt/mTOR pathway is essential for protein synthesis, autophagy, and cell proliferation. It has been discovered that berberine modifies this pathway, causing mTOR signaling to be inhibited and autophagy to be induced. This may have consequences for a number of illnesses, such as cancer, neurological diseases, and metabolic disorders.

It is important to remember that berberine's effects on cellular signaling pathways might vary depending on the cell type, dosage, and length of therapy. The interaction and crosstalk between these channels further complicate the overall effects of berberine.

Understanding how berberine affects various cellular signaling pathways sheds light on its possible therapeutic uses. The specific molecular processes and subsequent effects of berberine on these pathways in various illness situations, however, still need additional study.

2. Inhibition of Enzymes

The process through which a chemical, in this example berberine, interferes with an enzyme's activity and reduces its catalytic function is known as enzyme inhibition. It has been discovered that berberine has inhibitory effects on a number of enzymes, which have a variety of physiological consequences. The effects of berberine's inhibition of several enzymes will be covered in this article.

Inhibition of Acetylcholinesterase (AChE):

Acetylcholinesterase, an enzyme that breaks down the neurotransmitter acetylcholine, has been demonstrated to be inhibited by berberine. Berberine enhances cholinergic neurotransmission by increasing the concentration of acetylcholine in the synaptic cleft by inhibiting AChE. The setting of neurodegenerative diseases like Alzheimer's disease, where the breakdown of acetylcholine is accelerated, makes this inhibition of special relevance. By boosting cholinergic signaling, berberine's AChE inhibitory action may help slow cognitive decline.

Inhibition of Monoamine Oxidase (MAO):

Dopamine, norepinephrine, and serotonin are monoamine neurotransmitters, and monoamine oxidase is an enzyme involved in their metabolism. It has been discovered that berberine inhibits both MAO-A and MAO-B isoforms. Berberine may have antidepressant and neuroprotective effects by making these neurotransmitters more readily available by inhibiting MAO. However, it's crucial to remember that MAO inhibition might potentially cause negative effects and interact with certain drugs, so care should be taken.

preventing protein kinase:
Protein kinases such as protein kinase C (PKC) and mitogen-activated protein kinases (MAPKs) like ERK and JNK have been demonstrated to be inhibited by berberine. These protein kinases control cellular signaling pathways that control activities including cell division, growth, and inflammation. These kinases may be inhibited by berberine, which may explain why it has anti-inflammatory, anti-proliferative, and anti-cancer effects.

Blocking HMG-CoA Reductase:
According to some reports, the rate-limiting enzyme in the manufacture of

cholesterol, 3-hydroxy-3-methylglutaryl-coenzyme A (HMG-CoA) reductase, is inhibited by berberine. This inhibition causes a reduction in the production of cholesterol and an increase in the expression of the low-density lipoprotein receptor (LDLR), which aids in the removal of LDL cholesterol from circulation. The HMG-CoA reductase inhibitory action of berberine adds to its ability to decrease cholesterol and may be useful in treating dyslipidemia.

Inhibition of cyclooxygenase (COX):
Prostaglandins and other inflammatory mediators are produced by the enzyme cyclooxygenase, which berberine has shown to block. The anti-inflammatory characteristics of berberine and its potential application in treating inflammatory disorders may be attributed to this inhibition.

It is crucial to keep in mind that the precise processes and level of enzyme inhibition by berberine may change based on elements including concentration, exposure time, and the particular enzyme targeted. Additionally, since berberine may change how some drugs are metabolized and eliminated from the body, it may have an impact on drug interactions. Therefore, if using berberine together with other drugs, it is important to seek advice from a healthcare provider or pharmacist.

3. Effects of Antioxidants

Tinospora cordifolia contains the bioactive chemical berberine, which is known for its powerful antioxidant properties. Antioxidants are essential for defending the body against oxidative stress, which is linked to the generation of free radicals and reactive oxygen species (ROS). Multiple methods help berberine exhibit its antioxidant properties, which may have a positive impact on your health.

Free radical scavenger: Superoxide anions, hydroxyl radicals, and hydrogen peroxide are among the free radicals that berberine directly scavenges. Berberine assists in reducing the risk of oxidative harm to cells and tissues by neutralizing these highly reactive chemicals.

Enhancing Antioxidant Defense Systems: It has been shown that berberine increases the function of the body's natural antioxidant defense systems, which include enzymes like glutathione peroxidase (GPx), catalase, and superoxide dismutase (SOD). These enzymes are essential for neutralizing ROS and maintaining the redox equilibrium of cells.

Cellular Signaling Pathways: Berberine affects a number of cellular signaling pathways that are involved in inflammation and oxidative damage. The expression of antioxidant enzymes is regulated by the nuclear factor erythroid 2-related factor 2 (Nrf2) pathway, which supports cellular antioxidant defenses.

Berberine assists in preventing lipid peroxidation, which takes place when free radicals attack and damage the lipids in cell membranes. Berberine aids in maintaining the structural integrity and practicality of cell membranes by avoiding lipid peroxidation.

Reducing Inflammation: Oxidative stress and chronic inflammation are intimately related. By preventing the synthesis of pro-inflammatory cytokines and lowering the activation of inflammatory pathways, berberine has been demonstrated to have anti-inflammatory effects. Berberine indirectly boosts antioxidant defenses by lowering ROS generation through decreasing inflammation.

Berberine's antioxidant properties are crucial for preventing oxidative stress, but they also have consequences for a number of medical disorders. Numerous chronic illnesses, such as cancer, diabetes, cancer, and cardiovascular diseases, are thought to be caused by oxidative stress. Berberine may aid in preventing certain illnesses and promoting general health by exerting its antioxidant properties.

It is important to remember that berberine has antioxidant properties that are not only linked to Tinospora cordifolia but are shown in a variety of plant sources. Depending on the source and formulation of berberine employed, different antioxidant concentrations and modes of action may be present.

Before utilizing berberine, like with any dietary supplement or therapeutic substance, it is crucial to speak with a healthcare provider, particularly if you have any underlying medical issues or are on medication. They may provide advice on the right dose, possible interactions, and if berberine is a good fit for your particular requirements.

4. Modification of Gene Expression

The potential health advantages of berberine, a bioactive chemical present in several plants including Berberis species and Coptis chinensis, have been thoroughly investigated. The capacity of berberine to modify gene expression, affecting the activity of several genes involved in crucial biological processes, is one of the substance's interesting properties. The effect of berberine on gene expression and the underlying processes will be discussed in this article.

Regulation of Transcription Factors: Transcription factors are proteins that bind to DNA and regulate the expression of certain genes. Berberine has been shown to interact with and regulate a number of transcription factors. For instance, it has been shown that berberine activates the AMP-activated protein kinase (AMPK) pathway, a cellular energy sensor, which in turn controls the activity of several transcription factors involved in inflammation, metabolism, and other activities. Berberine activates AMPK, which has downstream effects on gene expression that include enhanced glucose metabolism, higher fatty acid oxidation, and reduced lipid synthesis.

Modulation of Epigenetic Factors: Epigenetic alterations, such as DNA methylation and histone modifications, are essential for controlling the expression of genes. It has been discovered that berberine affects these epigenetic elements, changing the patterns of gene expression. For instance, it has been shown that the methylation status of certain genes is impacted by berberine's ability to block DNA methyltransferases, which are the enzymes responsible for DNA methylation. Berberine may affect the expression of genes linked to numerous disorders, including cancer, through changing DNA methylation patterns.

Nuclear receptor activation: It has been shown that berberine interacts with nuclear receptors, which are proteins that control gene expression in response to certain ligands. For instance, the farnesoid X receptor (FXR), a nuclear receptor implicated in lipid homeostasis, inflammation, and bile acid metabolism, may be activated by berberine. Target genes involved in these pathways alter in expression as a result of berberine activating FXR. Peroxisome proliferator-activated receptor gamma

(PPAR gamma), a nuclear receptor involved in adipogenesis and glucose metabolism, has also been discovered to be activated by berberine.

Modulation of Signaling Pathways: By altering the activity of numerous signaling pathways involved in cellular functions, berberine may also have an impact on gene expression. For instance, berberine has been shown to inhibit the phosphoinositide 3-kinase (PI3K)/Akt pathway and the mitogen-activated protein kinase (MAPK) pathway, both of which are crucial for the growth, survival, and inflammation of cells. Berberine may affect the expression of genes involved in cell proliferation, death, and immunological responses by controlling these pathways.

MicroRNA regulation: MicroRNAs (miRNAs) are short non-coding RNAs that attach to messenger RNA (mRNA) and either prevent or promote translation of the mRNA, depending on the miRNA's target. It has been discovered that berberine modifies the expression of certain miRNAs, which in turn affects the expression of their target genes. For instance, it has been shown that berberine upregulates miR-122, a miRNA implicated in lipid metabolism, altering the expression of genes involved in the metabolism of fatty acids and cholesterol.

These are a few of the ways that berberine affects gene expression. Berberine may have significant impacts on gene expression patterns through interacting with transcription factors, epigenetic factors, nuclear receptors, signaling pathways, and miRNAs. These interactions eventually affect cellular functions and contribute to berberine's possible health advantages. To completely comprehend the nuances of berberine's effects on gene expression and its consequences for human health, further investigation is still required.

5. Induction of Autophagy

An essential part of cellular homeostasis maintenance and the elimination of damaged or superfluous components is the natural cellular process known as autophagy. The creation of autophagosomes, double-membrane structures, includes the breakdown and recycling of cellular components. Autophagy is regarded as a protective process that aids in cell survival, energy balance maintenance, and stress adaptation.

Numerous studies have shown that the natural substance berberine, which is present in many plants, including the Berberis species, may stimulate autophagy. Berberine's potential therapeutic benefits may be significantly impacted by the stimulation of autophagy. Here are some crucial details about the connection between berberine and the induction of autophagy:

Activation of AMP-activated protein kinase (AMPK): Autophagy and other metabolic processes, notably AMP-activated protein kinase (AMPK), are regulated by AMPK, which berberine has been discovered to stimulate. The key negative regulator of autophagy, the mammalian target of the rapamycin (mTOR) pathway, is inhibited as a result of berberine's stimulation of AMPK. Berberine accelerates the start of autophagy by blocking mTOR.

Modulation of autophagy-related proteins: Changing the expression and activity of important autophagy-related proteins is possible with berberine. It has been shown to increase the expression of the autophagy-starting protein beclin-1. Additionally, berberine promotes the transformation of LC3-I into LC3-II, which is crucial for the production of autophagosomes. The development and induction of the autophagic process are aided by these actions.

Protein aggregation clearance: Berberine has reportedly been shown to improve the clearance of protein aggregates linked to a variety of neurological disorders. Such disorders are characterized by the buildup of misfolded proteins, and defective autophagy may play a role in their development. Berberine may slow the course of illness by facilitating the clearance of protein aggregates via the induction of autophagy.

Protection from oxidative stress: Berberine has antioxidant capabilities and may reduce the harm caused by oxidative stress. Autophagy is one of the biological processes that oxidative stress may impair. Berberine stimulates autophagy by preserving the appropriate operation of cellular elements involved in the autophagic process by lowering oxidative stress.

Cancer cell death and tumor suppression: Berberine has been linked to both tumor suppression and cancer cell death via the stimulation of autophagy. Excessive autophagy in cancer cells may result in autophagic cell death, a kind of programmed cell death. This cell death process may be triggered by berberine-induced autophagy, which would eliminate cancer cells. Additionally, the autophagy-inducing features of berberine may contribute to its capacity to reduce tumor development and spread.

Even though berberine may activate autophagy, it's vital to remember that autophagy regulation can be complicated and context-dependent. Depending on the cell type, illness state, and other variables, the results of autophagy induction may differ. The specific mechanisms and therapeutic implications of berberine-induced autophagy in various situations still need more study.

In conclusion, it has been shown that berberine induces autophagy via a variety of pathways, such as activation of AMPK, modification of proteins involved in autophagy, removal of protein aggregates, defense against oxidative stress, and stimulation of cancer cell death. Our knowledge of the potential therapeutic uses of berberine in a variety of illnesses and ailments benefits from understanding the link between berberine and autophagy induction.

Berberine Safety and Side Effects

The natural substance berberine, which is present in a number of plants, has drawn interest due to its alleged health advantages. Although berberine is often seen to be safe when taken properly, it's crucial to be informed of any possible side effects and safety measures. Here are some crucial details about the security and negative consequences of berberine:

Generally Well-Tolerated: Berberine has been used for generations in traditional medicine with little to no negative side effects. The majority of people tolerate berberine well when they take it in the prescribed amounts. Individual reactions, however, may differ, and some individuals can have negative consequences.

Gastrointestinal Disturbances: The gastrointestinal side effects of berberine are the most often reported ones. These include gas, bloating, stomach discomfort, diarrhea, and constipation. These adverse effects are often modest and momentary, and they normally go away when the body becomes used to berberine. To reduce the danger of gastrointestinal side effects, starting with a smaller dosage and gradually increasing it is advised.

Drug Interactions: Certain drugs, notably those processed by the liver's cytochrome P450 enzymes, may interact with berberine. It could have an impact on how these enzymes function and how well certain medications are metabolized and eliminated from the body. Increased medication levels and associated negative consequences may result from this. Before using berberine, it is advised to speak with a healthcare provider if you are already taking any drugs, particularly those that are processed by the liver.

nursing: There is little evidence available on the safety of berberine while nursing or during pregnancy. As a result, it is often advised to abstain from using berberine during these times in order to be safe.

Before using Berberine in such circumstances, it is crucial to speak with a healthcare provider.

Blood Pressure and Blood Glucose: Berberine has been demonstrated to reduce blood pressure and blood sugar levels. Those who have diabetes or hypertension may benefit from this, although they could need to change their drug amounts. It's crucial to routinely check your blood sugar and blood pressure levels if you have diabetes or hypertension and are thinking about taking berberine. You should also speak with your healthcare practitioner about the best course of action.

Liver and Kidney Function: In certain people, berberine has been linked to moderate increases in liver enzyme levels. It is advised to use caution and speak with a doctor before taking berberine if you have underlying liver issues. Additionally, because the kidneys are the main organs via which berberine is removed, those with compromised renal function should be careful and speak with their doctor.

Allergic Reactions: Although uncommon, allergic responses to berberine have been documented. After using berberine, if you have symptoms like a rash, itching, swelling, lightheadedness, or trouble breathing, stop using it right away and get medical help.

It is crucial to remember that berberine's safety and negative effects might change based on the user, the dose, and the length of usage. It is advised to speak with a healthcare provider before beginning berberine supplementation in order to assure safety and reduce possible hazards, particularly if you have any underlying medical issues or are on medication.

Formulas and Berberine Dosage

There are many formulations of berberine, a natural substance with possible health advantages, that may be taken as a supplement. Depending on the particular health problem being treated, berberine may need a different formulation and dose. Here are some typical berberine formulations and dose recommendations:

Available Berberine Forms

A natural substance called berberine, which has a number of health advantages, may be taken as a supplement in a variety of ways. These alternatives allow people to choose the most practical and appropriate way to take berberine. The following are some typical dosages of berberine:

pills and Capsules: Berberine is often available in pills or capsules. These formulations, which are housed in a gelatin or veggie capsule or compacted into a tablet, include berberine in a powdered form, often in the form of a standardized extract. Tablets and capsules are practical and provide accurate dosage. The usual way to take them is by mouth with water and the prescribed dose.

Liquid Extracts: Berberine is furthermore offered in liquid extract form. Concentrated berberine is dissolved in a liquid basis, such as glycerin or alcohol, in liquid extracts. They could include a dropper or measurement tool to make administration simple. Liquid extracts may be combined with water or other liquids for ingestion and give flexibility in dose modification.

Topical Creams or Gels: Some berberine formulations are made for use topically. These creams or gels are applied directly to the skin and include berberine as an active component. Skin infections and other dermatological disorders are often treated with topical berberine preparations. They should be used in accordance with the manufacturer's instructions or a healthcare professional's recommendation.

Combination Formulations: Berberine is often used in combination formulations. These formulations could also include vitamins, minerals, or complementary substances that combine with berberine to assist certain health objectives. Examples include berberine preparations that target blood sugar control or berberine combinations with other herbs for digestive assistance. Depending on the particular product, the ingredients list, and dose recommendations may change.

It is important to note that depending on the brand and location, various berberine forms may not always be readily available. It is best to stick with trusted brands and carefully study product labels to learn about the precise form, concentration and advised dose.

It is crucial to take into consideration personal tastes, practicality, and elements like ease of administration and absorption while choosing the right type of berberine. The best form and dose of berberine should be chosen depending on specific health requirements and objectives; this should be done in consultation with a healthcare expert or a competent herbalist.

Berberine dosage that is suggested

The right amount of berberine to take depends on the ailment being treated, as well as personal characteristics including age, weight, and general health. Here are some broad dose suggestions for berberine, however, it's crucial to speak with a doctor for specific advice:

Blood Glucose Management: A common dose range for those looking to promote healthy blood glucose levels is 500-1500 mg of berberine per day. You may spread this out across two or three doses over the day. For the best dose adjustment, it is advised to start with a lower dosage and raise it gradually while monitoring blood glucose levels and seeking expert advice.

Cardiovascular Health: A typical dose range for berberine is 900–1500 mg per day to promote cardiovascular health and maintain healthy cholesterol levels. You may split this up into two or three doses. Once again, it's crucial to consult a medical expert when deciding on the right dose depending on each patient's requirements and to keep an eye on how it affects lipid profiles.

Digestive Health: A normal dose range for berberine is 300–600 mg per day for digestive support, including fostering a healthy gut microbiota and treating gastrointestinal symptoms. You may split this up into two doses. To get tailored dose recommendations, it is advised to speak with a healthcare expert since individual reactions may differ.

Weight control: Berberine's possible usefulness in weight control has been researched. Typically, 500 mg should be taken three times a day, an hour before meals, for this reason. However, it is essential to collaborate with a medical expert or a licensed dietitian to create a thorough weight-management strategy and guarantee its safe and efficient use.

Other Medical issues: Different dosages may be advised for those with other medical issues such as liver support, immune system modulation, or antibacterial actions. It is crucial to get advice from a medical expert who can evaluate unique health requirements and provide dose recommendations depending on the intended therapeutic result.

A healthcare practitioner must be consulted before beginning berberine supplementation, particularly if you are taking other drugs or have underlying medical issues, since berberine may interfere with certain medications. The right dose, possible interactions, and monitoring for effectiveness and safety may all be covered by them.

Depending on the health issue being treated, different berberine dosages may be advised. Although broad dose ranges are given, it is crucial to speak with a healthcare provider for more specific dosage advice. To guarantee safe and efficient use for the best health results, they may consider individual circumstances, evaluate possible combinations, and track the effects of berberine.

Therapies in Combination with Berberine

A natural substance called berberine, which has a variety of positive health effects, may be used in conjunction with other treatments to boost their potency or treat certain medical disorders. Berberine may have synergistic benefits when combined with alternative therapies or lifestyle changes, which can improve health results. Here are several instances of berberine-based combination therapies:

Metabolic health: For illnesses like type 2 diabetes or metabolic syndrome, berberine is often administered in conjunction with lifestyle therapies. Berberine may help increase insulin sensitivity, control blood sugar levels, and maintain healthy lipid profiles when used in conjunction with regular exercise, a balanced diet, and weight management techniques.

Cardiovascular Health: Berberine may be included in a whole strategy for cardiovascular health that also includes dietary changes, consistent exercise, and medicines (if needed). Berberine combined with dietary modifications and conventional therapies may maintain healthy blood pressure, lower cholesterol levels, and improve overall heart health.

Gut Health: Berberine is beneficial for gut health due to its antibacterial and anti-inflammatory characteristics. It may assist in restoring a healthy balance of gut flora, lowering inflammation in the gut, and improving digestive well-being when taken in conjunction with probiotics or other gut-supporting products.

Weight control: Berberine's possible usefulness in weight control has been researched. Supplementing with berberine while following a calorie-restricted diet, getting regular exercise, and using behavior modification techniques may assist long-term weight management and help weight reduction attempts.

Combinations of herbs: To treat certain health issues, berberine may sometimes be combined with other herbs. For instance, berberine is often used with herbs like Coptis chinensis or Scutellaria baicalensis in traditional Chinese medicine for their synergistic benefits in treating digestive issues or promoting liver function.

It is essential to speak with a certified herbal medicine practitioner or a healthcare professional before adopting berberine-based combination therapy. Based on individual health requirements, probable interactions, and the best combinations for certain medical situations, they may provide tailored suggestions.

While combination treatments may have advantages, it is crucial to use them safely and effectively by adhering to dose guidelines, keeping an eye out for any possible interactions or adverse effects, and communicating with medical specialists.

Berberine's therapeutic benefits may be improved and health results can be optimized by combining it with other treatments, lifestyle changes, or herbal medicines. The best combination of treatments, dosages, and monitoring for best outcomes must be determined in consultation with a healthcare practitioner whether the herb is taken for weight management, metabolic health, cardiovascular health, gut health, or in conjunction with other herbs.

Future Prospects and Berberine Research Directions

Due to its conceivable health advantages, berberine, a natural substance with a long history of traditional usage, has drawn considerable interest in contemporary scientific study. Several new views and research axes arise as we dive further into understanding its mechanisms of action and therapeutic uses. Here are some potential areas for berberine research in the future:

Clinical Trials and Evidence-Based Research: Although preclinical research and observational data suggest that berberine may be useful, more carefully planned clinical trials are required to determine the drug's efficacy, safety, and ideal doses for a range of medical disorders. Berberine will become a common treatment choice if randomized controlled trials (RCTs) are conducted with greater sample numbers and longer durations.

Mechanistic Insights: Despite tremendous advancements in our knowledge of the processes behind berberine's therapeutic effects, there is still more to learn. The specific molecular mechanisms by which berberine acts must yet be clarified, especially in complicated illnesses including cancer, metabolic problems, and neurodegenerative ailments. Modern methods including systems biology methodologies and omics technologies (genomics, proteomics, and metabolomics) may provide important insights into the complex processes of berberine.

Pharmacokinetics and Drug Delivery Systems: To maximize the therapeutic potential of berberine, it is crucial to understand its pharmacokinetics, which includes its absorption, distribution, metabolism, and excretion. Its effectiveness may be increased by creating novel drug delivery methods that boost berberine's bioavailability and target certain tissues or cells. The pharmacokinetic profile and targeted distribution of berberine may be improved using nanoparticles, liposomes, and other nanotechnology-based strategies.

Combination Therapies: Investigating the synergistic effects of berberine when combined with other substances or traditional therapies may lead to the development of novel therapeutic approaches. Combination medicines that improve therapeutic results and reduce side effects may be found by looking into possible interactions between berberine and pharmaceutical pharmaceuticals. In addition to optimizing dose schedules, these investigations may provide light on the underlying processes of interactions.

Personalized medicine: Since berberine responses may differ from person to person, further study is required to find any biomarkers or hereditary components that might affect the effectiveness and security of berberine. Healthcare providers will be able to customize berberine treatment programs based on an individual's genetic and phenotypic traits by developing predictive models and putting personalized medicine strategies into practice, which will lead to better results.

Formulation Optimization: Berberine is available in a variety of formulations, although research is still being done to optimize the drug's delivery methods to increase bioavailability, stability, and patient compliance. Berberine's solubility, absorption, and sustained release may be improved using novel formulation methods such as nanoemulsions, microencapsulations, and prodrug strategies, making it more beneficial and practical for patients.

Safety and Long-Term Effects: More study is required to fully comprehend the long-term safety profile of berberine, especially at larger dosages or during continuous use. The safety of berberine will be better understood by looking at possible side effects, and drug interactions, and monitoring the effects on important organs like the liver and kidneys. This will also assist set rules for the proper and responsible use of berberine.

Comparative Studies: Comparing berberine with other traditional treatments or herbal substances used for related medical diseases might provide light on how effective, safe, and cost-efficient it is in comparison. The relative advantages and hazards of berberine in comparison to alternative therapy choices may be better understood by healthcare professionals and patients via the conduct of head-to-head studies and systematic reviews/meta-analyses.

Translational research and clinical guidelines: For berberine to be widely used as a therapeutic agent, the gap between fundamental research and clinical practice must be closed. The establishment of evidence-based clinical recommendations for the use of berberine may be facilitated by collaborative efforts involving researchers, clinicians, regulatory bodies, and legislators, assuring its safe and efficient incorporation into standard medical practice.

In conclusion, berberine research has a very bright future. To further our knowledge of berberine's therapeutic potential, more clinical trials, mechanistic research, pharmacokinetic investigations, and personalized medicine strategies are required. Its therapeutic value will be increased by enhancing drug delivery methods, investigating combination treatments, and guaranteeing long-term safety. We may realize the full potential of berberine as a beneficial natural component for enhancing human health and well-being by tackling these study objectives.

Conclusion

The natural substance berberine has a long history and a wide range of medicinal applications. It has been historically utilized as a medicine in many different cultures, and contemporary scientific study has shed light on its methods of action and health advantages. Numerous pharmacological actions of berberine include anti-inflammatory, antioxidant, antibacterial, and anti-cancer properties.

Plants including Coptis chinensis, Berberis vulgaris, Berberis aristata, Hydrastis canadensis, Mahonia aquifolium, and Tinospora cordifolia are sources of berberine. These plants are important natural sources of berberine and have long been used in traditional medical systems.

A number of cellular signaling pathways, including AMP-activated protein kinase (AMPK), insulin signaling, and inflammatory pathways, are modulated by Berberine as part of its mechanisms of action. It has positive impacts on a variety of medical issues, including blood glucose control, immunological support, cardiovascular health, digestive health, and weight management, by affecting many targets inside cells.

Although berberine has potential as a natural remedy, it is vital to think about its safety and any adverse effects. Although adverse responses are relatively uncommon, combinations with other drugs and excessive doses might cause moderate side effects including nausea or diarrhea. Before beginning berberine supplementation, particularly for those with underlying medical disorders or those who use drugs, it is crucial to speak with a healthcare practitioner.

There are several different ways to get berberine, including pills, capsules, liquid extracts, lotions for the skin, and mixed formulations. The best form to use will depend on your personal preferences, your convenience, and the particular health issue you're trying to treat.

Future research should focus on enhancing drug delivery mechanisms, discovering combination therapy, performing well-designed clinical trials, and developing personalized medicine strategies in order to fully fulfill Berberine's promise. The use of berberine in healthcare will be improved further through comparative research, long-term safety analyses, and the creation of evidence-based clinical recommendations.

In conclusion, berberine is a natural substance with a lengthy history and wide-ranging medicinal potential. It is an effective tool for enhancing health and well-being due to its wide range of health benefits, methods of action, and availability in a variety of forms. We can unleash the full potential of berberine and exploit its advantages for those looking for natural and holistic approaches to healthcare by continuing to investigate its uses and conducting rigorous scientific studies.

Term Glossary

Berberine: The natural substance berberine, which is present in many plants, is well-known for its wide range of medicinal advantages.

AMP-activated protein kinase (AMPK): The enzyme AMP-activated protein kinase (AMPK) is essential for maintaining the equilibrium of cellular energy. Berberine activates AMPK, which has a variety of positive effects on metabolism and health.

Insulin signaling: The route via which insulin controls cellular functions such as glucose metabolism is known as insulin signaling. It has been shown that berberine alters insulin signaling, which helps in controlling blood sugar.

Antioxidant: A chemical that aids in the body's defense against damaging free radicals, lowering oxidative stress and shielding cells from deterioration.

Anti-inflammatory: Capable of reducing inflammation, which is often a contributing cause of many chronic illnesses.

Antimicrobial: Substances that prevent the development or eradication of microorganisms like fungi, viruses, and bacteria.

Anticancer: Possesses qualities that aid in preventing or restraining the development of cancer cells.

Pharmacokinetics: Pharmacokinetics is the study of how a drug enters the body, is distributed throughout it, is processed, and then is eliminated.

Drug Delivery Systems: Systems for delivering drugs or therapeutic substances to the body's intended locations are known as drug delivery systems.

Randomized controlled trial (RCT): An RCT is a form of scientific research in which participants are randomly allocated to various treatment groups in order to evaluate the efficacy of a given intervention or therapy.

Biomarkers: Biomarkers are quantifiable indicators used to assess biological processes, disease development, and therapeutic response.

Personalized Medicine: Personalized medicine is a medical treatment strategy that adjusts to a patient's unique traits, including genetics, way of life, and environmental influences.

Nanoparticles: To increase medication stability, bioavailability, and targeted administration, drug delivery systems often utilize nanoparticles, tiny particles with diameters on the nanoscale.

Liposomes: Liposomes are synthetic lipid bilayer-based vesicles that are employed as medication delivery vehicles.

Prodrug: A substance that is either inert or hardly active but is transformed into an active drug in the body by metabolic processes.

Comparative Studies: Studies that contrast the efficacy, safety, or other characteristics of several methods or forms of therapy are known as comparative studies.

Systematic Review: A systematic review is a thorough and organized examination of the body of knowledge in a field of study, often comprising data synthesis and statistical analysis.

Meta-analysis: A statistical study known as a meta-analysis integrates data from several separate research to get more solid and trustworthy conclusions.

Translational research: The process of bridging the gap between scientific discoveries (basic research) and their implementation in clinical practice.

Evidence-based clinical guidelines: Clinical recommendations for healthcare professionals are based on the most up-to-date scientific data with the goal of assisting in clinical decision-making and enhancing patient outcomes.

Abbreviations list

AMP-activated protein kinase - AMPK
Randomized controlled trial - (RCT)
Body mass index, - BMI
Low-density lipoprotein - LDL
High-density lipoprotein - HDL
Hemoglobin A1c - HbA1c
Reactive oxygen species - (ROS)
Tumor necrosis factor - (TNF)
Interleukin - (IL)
Reactive protein - CRP
Low-density lipoprotein cholesterol - (LDL-C)
High-density lipoprotein cholesterol - (HDL-C)
Bone mineral density - (BMD)
Central nervous system - (CNS)
GI stands for digestive.
Peroxisome proliferator-activated receptor - PPAR.
Protein kinase C - PKC
Nuclear factor-kappa B - (NF-B)
SRT - Sirtuin
Type 2 diabetes - T2D